Essential workouts for improving stability
and overall wellness

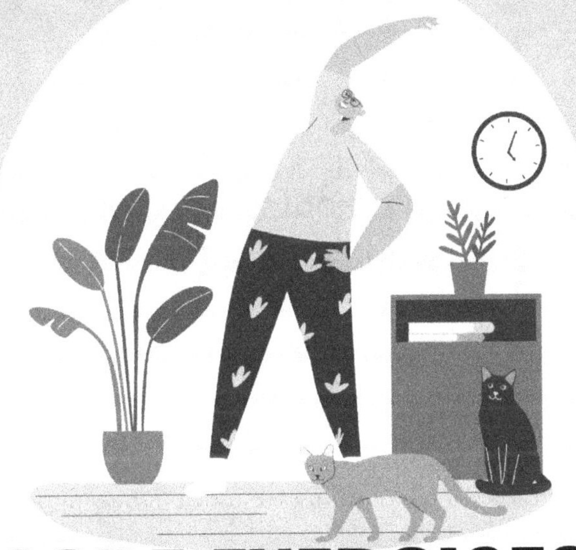

CORE EXERCISES
FOR SENIORS

Dr. Bryant D Baldwin

Core Exercises for seniors

Essential Workouts for Improving Stability and Overall Wellness

Dr Bryant D Baldwin

Table of contents

Introduction

One key part of overall physical health for seniors is a strong and stable core. The core, which encompasses the muscles in your belly, back, hips, and pelvis, serves as the foundation for your body's mobility and stability. It plays a key part in everyday actions such as walking, standing, sitting, bending, and lifting, as well as in maintaining excellent balance and posture.

In this book, ***"Core Exercises for Seniors: Essential workouts for improving stability and overall wellness"*** we will discuss the importance of core strength for seniors and present a thorough guide to effective core exercises specifically developed for older folks.

Whether you are a senior trying to increase your core strength, a caregiver aiding a loved one, or a fitness expert working with older clients, this book will provide you with essential ideas and practical exercises to help you achieve your goals.

With clear instructions, images, and variations for various fitness levels, this book is suited for seniors of all abilities, from those who are just starting their fitness journey to those who are more active and looking to develop their core strength.

The exercises contained in this book are safe, and effective, and may be performed at home or in a gym setting with minimum equipment. They can be simply implemented into your routine to help you increase your core strength, boost your balance and stability, lower the risk of falls, and promote total functional fitness.

In addition to the physical benefits, strengthening your core can also have good consequences on your mental well-being. By enhancing your physical strength and stability, you may boost your self-confidence, enhance your mood, and increase your entire quality of life.

So, whether you are wanting to maintain your independence, increase your physical performance, or simply boost your general well-being as a senior, *"Core Exercises for Seniors: Essential workouts for improving stability and overall wellness"* is the right guide to help you on your fitness journey.

Let's begin on this amazing journey together and find the strength that resides within you!

Importance Of Core Strength For Elders

Core strength is vital for seniors as it plays a fundamental role in maintaining general health, stability, and mobility. The core muscles, including the muscles of the belly, lower back, hips, and pelvis, establish the foundation for all motions and offer stability to the spine and other joints. Here are some important reasons why core strength is essential for seniors:

1. Balance and Fall Prevention

As seniors age, their balance may become disturbed, leading to an increased risk of falls and injuries. Strong core muscles help preserve balance and stability, minimizing the risk of falls and enhancing general safety and quality of life.

2. Posture and Spinal Health

Core muscles provide support to the spine and assist maintain appropriate posture. Weak core muscles can lead to poor posture and raise the chance of developing disorders such as kyphosis (hunchback) or lordosis (swayback), which can cause pain and discomfort.

3. Functional Mobility

Core strength is crucial for performing daily activities such as getting up from a chair, bending down to pick up objects, and reaching aloft. Improved core strength can enhance functional mobility and independence in seniors, allowing them to keep their capacity to complete daily duties.

4. Muscle and Joint Health

Strong core muscles assist the transfer of the load uniformly across the joints, lowering stress on the joints and minimizing the risk of developing joint pain and arthritis.

5. Breathing and Digestion

The diaphragm, which is a primary muscle involved in breathing, is part of the core muscular group. Strong core muscles help boost respiratory function, which is vital for seniors' general health. Additionally, core strength helps assist in appropriate digestion and bowel function.

6. Enhanced Sports and Physical Activities

For seniors who wish to engage in sports or physical activities such as gardening, golfing, or swimming, core strength is vital for stability, balance, and efficient movement.

7. Pain Management

Core strengthening exercises can help treat chronic illnesses such as low back pain, which is common among seniors. Strengthening the muscles around the spine can give stability and decrease pain.

Benefits of Core Exercises

Core exercises are an important component of a well-rounded fitness routine, as they provide several benefits for overall health and well-being. Some of the benefits of core exercises include:

1. Better Core Strength

The primary advantage of core exercises is better core strength. Your core muscles, including your abs, obliques, lower back, and pelvic floor, provide stability and support to your spine, pelvis, and hips. Strong core muscles help you maintain excellent posture, reduce the risk of lower back pain, and boost your ability to perform useful motions in daily life and other physical activities.

2. Enhanced Stability and Balance

Core workouts can enhance your stability and balance by strengthening the muscles that support your body's center of gravity. This can help reduce the chance of falls and injuries, particularly in older persons or athletes engaged in sports that involve balance, such as yoga, gymnastics, or martial arts.

3. Better Athletic Performance

A strong core is crucial for good athletic performance. Core workouts can assist athletes to create power and move energy efficiently between their upper and lower body, boosting their performance in sports like running, swimming, golfing, and weightlifting.

4. Improved Posture

Core workouts can help you achieve better posture by strengthening the muscles that support your spine and pelvis. This can help you keep an upright posture and prevent the danger of slouching or hunching, which can lead to poor posture and musculoskeletal imbalances over time.

5. Reduced Risk of Lower Back Discomfort

Core exercises are particularly good at strengthening the muscles that support the lower back, which can help reduce the risk of lower back discomfort. A strong core helps stabilize the spine and maintain good alignment, decreasing the pressure on the lower back during regular activities or heavy lifting.

6. Functional Fitness

Core exercises focus on strengthening the strength and stability of your core muscles, which are involved in practically every movement you undertake in daily life, such as bending, lifting, twisting, and reaching. By strengthening your core, you can boost your ability to perform these functional actions safely and efficiently.

7. Better Breathing and Digestion

Core exercises also engage the diaphragm, which is a crucial muscle involved in breathing, and the muscles of the pelvic floor, which are important for appropriate digestion and bladder control. Strengthening these muscles can lead to improved respiratory patterns and better digestion.

Chapter 1

Understanding Core Muscles

Maintaining general physical health and practical movement requires strong core muscles. However, a lot of people are erroneous in thinking that the core is just made up of the abdominal muscles, sometimes known as the "six-pack."

In actuality, the core is a complex collection of muscles that support, stabilize, and coordinate the spine and pelvis. To perform at your best, avoid injuries, and enhance daily activities, it is essential to comprehend the true nature of your core muscles and their function in the body.

In this chapter, we'll go deep into the inner workings of the core muscles, learning about their anatomy, purpose, and significance in everything from sports and fitness to everyday activities and posture.

What Muscles Make Up the Core?

The abdomen, lower back, pelvis, and hips are all parts of the body that have muscles that make up the core. These muscles serve as the body's structural support system and give the spine and pelvis stability and support. The several muscle groups that make up the core muscles include:

1. Rectus Abdominis

The most famous core muscle, also referred to as the "abs." The lengthy muscle that supports the trunk and runs vertically down the front of the abdomen is in charge of flexing the spine.

2. Deep within the belly, the transverse abdominis muscle serves as a corset, wrapping around the stomach and supporting the spine and pelvis.

3. The muscles known as the obliques, which run along the sides of the belly, are in charge of the spine's lateral flexion and rotation.

4. Small muscles called multifidus run along the spine and stabilize each vertebra, enabling optimal spinal alignment and movement.

5. Erector Spinae

These muscles go along the lower back and help to keep the spine extended and upright.

6. Pelvic Floor Muscles

These muscles are found at the base of the pelvis and are in charge of stabilizing the pelvis, supporting the organs in the pelvic cavity, and preserving fecal and urine continence.

How They Work

The body's stability, balance, and strength are provided by the coordinated action of the core muscles. Together, they support the spine, pelvis, and hips through a variety of motions and activities. The core muscles cooperate in the following ways:

1. Stability

The core muscles cooperate to give the spine and pelvic stability, which is essential for preserving good posture and avoiding accidents. For instance, the core muscles activate during physical activity like running or jumping to stabilize the spine and pelvis, limiting excessive movement, and preserving normal alignment.

2. Balance

The core muscles are essential for keeping your balance and your coordination. They cooperate to keep the body's center of gravity stable, enabling fluid and precise motions. The core muscles contract to keep you balanced and prevent falls or accidents when you engage in balance-required activities like standing on one leg or executing yoga poses.

3. Functional motions

Almost all of the body's functional motions, such as bending, twisting, lifting, and reaching, utilize the core muscles. Together, they carry forces from the lower body to the upper body and vice versa, making actions possible that are effective and well-coordinated. For instance, the core muscles work to support the spine and pelvis when you bend over to pick something up off the ground. This enables you to lift the object safely.

4. Support for Posture

For the overall health of the spine, good posture must be maintained, which is the responsibility of the core muscles. Together, they support the spine and pelvis, preventing shoulder hunching or rounding, and preserving a neutral spine position. Maintaining a healthy spine and preventing back discomfort need good posture.

The muscles of the core are involved in breathing as well. The core muscles include the diaphragm, a dome-shaped muscle situated at the base of the ribcage. By contracting and relaxing to aid in inhaling and exhaling, it plays a critical part in the breathing process. To maintain correct intra-abdominal pressure while breathing, the diaphragm collaborates with other core muscles including the transverse abdominis and pelvic floor muscles. This stability of the core and support of effective respiratory function result from this process.

The Significance of Using your Core Muscles

The core muscles are essential for supporting the structure and operation of the human body, an engineering wonder. The abdominal, back, and pelvic muscles are among the core muscles, which are found in the body's trunk. Together, these muscles give the spine, pelvis, and internal organs stability, strength, and support. Not only is using the core muscles important for keeping excellent posture and avoiding back pain, but it also promotes general health and fitness.

All body movements are built on the foundation of the core muscles. Every movement we perform, whether it be bending, twisting, lifting, or reaching, involves the core muscles. They serve as stabilizers, giving the spine and pelvis, the body's primary hubs, support, and control. Poor posture, diminished stability, and an elevated risk of injury can result from weak or inactive core muscles.

The improvement of posture is one of the main advantages of using the core muscles. People who spend a lot of time sitting at computers or hunching over electronics tend to have poor posture due to their sedentary lifestyle. A slouched posture caused by weak core muscles can cause muscle imbalances, joint misalignments, and back pain. Maintaining a neutral spine position encourages healthy posture and lowers the likelihood of musculoskeletal problems. This is made possible by using the core muscles.

It's also crucial to contract the core muscles to prevent back pain. The back is stabilized by the core muscles, which also act as a natural corset to shield the spine from undue pressure and stress. Strong and active core muscles assist in evenly distributing the stress across the spine, lowering the possibility of painful overuse injuries. Additionally, strengthening the core muscles helps to realign the spine and relieve pressure on the intervertebral discs, which can help to ward off ailments like herniated discs and degenerative disc disease.

Engaging the core muscles is essential for increasing overall strength and fitness, as well as for supporting good posture and preventing back problems. From weightlifting to running to yoga, almost all exercises and physical activities require the core muscles. Greater strength, agility, and coordination are made possible by a strong core, which provides a solid foundation for movement. Additionally, it aids in the efficient transfer of force between the upper and lower bodies, facilitating actions that are more effective and efficient. Engaging the core muscles is crucial for optimizing performance and lowering the risk of injury when executing complex movements, heavier weightlifting, or running quicker.

Maintaining functional fitness is largely dependent on using the core muscles, especially as we become older. Our muscles, particularly our core muscles, tend to deteriorate as we age. The risk of falls and injuries may arise as a result of a reduction in balance, stability, and mobility. Maintaining core stability and strength, which are essential for carrying out daily activities like walking, standing, and getting up from a chair, can be accomplished by practicing exercises like planks, bridges, and rotational motions.

The core muscles may be worked in a variety of ways, and incorporating exercises that focus on various core muscles into your routine will help you receive a well-rounded core workout. Planks, which work the lower back, obliques, and deep stabilizing muscles, bridges, which work the glutes, hamstrings, and lower back muscles, and Russian twists, which work the obliques and transverse abdominis, are some exercises that are effective for working the core muscles.

It's vital to remember that properly activating your core muscles should be a part of all of your daily activities in addition to performing isolated core exercises. This entails keeping your spine in a neutral position during various exercises and activities, as well as maintaining good posture while sitting, standing, and walking. You may develop a strong and functional core by being mindful of your core muscles and purposefully using them throughout exercises and daily activities.

Chapter 2

Warm-Up Exercises That Are Safe And Effective

Seniors can lower their risk of falls and injuries by improving their balance, stability, and posture with core exercises that focus on the muscles of the belly, back, and pelvis. However, it's imperative to begin with a secure and efficient warm-up program before moving on to core workouts.

An effective warm-up gets the body ready for exercise, boosts blood flow to the muscles, and reduces the risk of injury. This chapter will examine a variety of warm-up exercises created especially for seniors to provide a secure and efficient beginning to their regular fitness program.

These warm-up exercises for seniors will help them loosen up, increase flexibility, and get ready for a satisfying and advantageous core workout. They range from moderate stretches to low-impact activities. Let's get started by learning how to correctly warm up for core exercises to maintain our bodies' strength and flexibility as we age.

Body Preparation for Core Exercises

Regular exercise is important for leading a healthy lifestylc, and seniors can benefit especially from core exercises. A solid core can lower the risk of falls and injuries while enhancing balance, stability, and posture. For seniors to ensure safe and efficient workouts, it's imperative to properly prepare their bodies before beginning core activities.

In this part, we'll look at the crucial procedures older citizens should follow to get their bodies ready for core exercises.

Seek advice from a healthcare expert
Seniors must speak with their healthcare provider before beginning any new fitness program, especially if they have any existing medical ailments or worries. Based on a person's current state of health, medical history, and degree of fitness, a healthcare practitioner can offer tailored suggestions and recommendations. Based on a person's particular circumstances, they can also assist in determining whether any special precautions or adaptations should be made for core activities.

1. Stretch and warm-up

Seniors should always warm up before exercising since it increases blood flow to the muscles, gets the body ready for physical activity, and lowers the risk of accidents. Seniors can warm up for five to ten minutes with light cardiovascular exercises like brisk walking or cycling before beginning their core fitness program. Stretching exercises should be performed after the warm-up to increase flexibility and mobility. Target key muscular groups such as the hamstrings, quadriceps, calves, shoulders, and back when stretching slowly without bouncing. Flexibility can be increased and the danger of muscular injuries decreased by holding each stretch for 15 to 30 seconds and repeating the exercise a few times.

2. Focus on proper posture

Seniors must maintain good posture during core exercises to enable efficient and secure workouts. Unnecessary tension on the neck, shoulders, and back from poor posture can result in pain or injuries. Seniors should concentrate on maintaining a neutral spine alignment, which entails keeping the spine's typical alignment of its natural curvature. This can be accomplished by using your core muscles during activity and avoiding hunching over, rounding your shoulders, or arching your back. Being mindful of your posture not only increases the efficiency of your core exercises but also helps you maintain better posture throughout the day, which lowers your chance of developing musculoskeletal problems.

3. Start with simple workouts.

Starting with fundamental exercises that are suitable for their fitness level and physical capabilities is vital for seniors who are new to core exercises or who have little experience with physical activity. Simple exercises like seated leg lifts, seated marches, and sit twists might be a good place to start to gradually engage the core muscles and increase strength. Seniors can progressively proceed to more difficult exercises like sitting Russian twists, plank variations, or bicycle crunches as they get stronger and feel more comfortable. To prevent strain or damage, it's crucial to move forward at a rate that seems safe and comfortable.

4. Remember to breathe

Even though they are sometimes disregarded, proper breathing techniques are essential for elderly citizens' core activities. The act of breathing keeps the abdominal muscles in place and guarantees that the body receives enough oxygen when exercising. When performing core exercises, seniors should concentrate on taking deep breaths through their noses and expelling gently through their mouths. It's vital to avoid holding your breath because doing so can strain your core muscles and raise intra-abdominal pressure. In addition to enhancing the efficiency of core exercises, proper breathing also encourages relaxation and eases physical strain.

5. Keep hydrated and pay attention to your body.

Seniors should drink plenty of water when exercising to avoid dehydration-related weariness and cramping. To stay adequately hydrated, seniors should drink water before, during, and after their main exercise program. During core workouts, it's also critical to pay attention to any discomfort or pain your body may be experiencing. It's critical to stop right away and get advice from a healthcare provider if something seems strange or hurts. Pushing through discomfort or pain can result in injuries, so it's better to err on the side of caution and alter workouts as necessary.

6. Add diversity and growth.

Seniors should include variation and advancement in their core training regimen to keep their core muscles challenged and progressing. Exercise's intensity, duration, or difficulty can be steadily increased over time to achieve this. Seniors can obtain a well-rounded core workout by experimenting with various exercises that target distinct core muscles, such as the rectus abdominis, obliques, and lower back. Tools like stability balls or resistance bands can be added to core exercises to increase variation and difficulty. The danger of accidents might be increased by rapid or drastic changes, therefore it's vital to advance gradually.

7. Maintain a healthy diet and sleep

The body must be well-fueled and rested to be ready for core activities. Seniors should make sure they are eating a balanced diet with enough protein, good fats, and carbohydrates to provide their muscles with the nutrition they need to grow and repair. Additionally, adequate rest and sleep are necessary for healthy energy levels, muscular repair, and general well-being. Seniors should prioritize rest days in between core exercise sessions and strive for 7-9 hours of excellent sleep each night to give their bodies time to heal and repair.

To ensure a safe and successful workout, elders must prepare their bodies for core exercises. Key steps in preparing the body for core exercises include speaking with a healthcare provider, warming up and stretching, maintaining good posture, beginning with simple exercises, concentrating on breathing, drinking plenty of water, listening to the body, incorporating variety and progression, and maintaining healthy nutrition and rest.

Vitality of Stretching

Stretching is frequently disregarded as a critical part of a healthy lifestyle, yet it is necessary to preserve general well-being. Stretching can have several positive effects on your physical and mental health, regardless of whether you are an athlete, a fitness enthusiast, or simply lead a sedentary lifestyle.

Stretching entails purposefully lengthening your muscles and tendons to promote flexibility, improve circulation, and improve performance. It goes beyond simply touching your toes or making a few arm circles. We'll talk about the value of stretching and why it should be a regular part of your daily routine in this post.

Flexibility, which is the range of motion in your joints, is essential for safely and effectively engaging in a variety of physical activities. By extending contracted muscles and enhancing joint mobility, regular stretching can assist to increase flexibility. You are less prone to strain or damage your muscles during physical activities like exercise, sports, or even regular duties like bending, reaching, and lifting when your muscles are more flexible. By preventing some muscles from getting too tight, which can result in muscular imbalances and postural problems, stretching also helps to preserve muscle balance.

Stretching is not only good for your physical health, but it also significantly contributes to your mental wellness. Muscle pain and tightness can result from stress and tension building up in the muscles. By encouraging relaxation and lowering stress, stretching can aid in releasing this tension.

The parasympathetic nervous system, the body's natural relaxation response, can be activated during stretching since it involves slow, deliberate motions and deep breathing. In addition to lowering blood pressure and pulse rate, this can aid in promoting calmness and relaxation.

Stretching might additionally help with posture and body awareness. A variety of musculoskeletal problems, including back pain, neck discomfort, and headaches, can be brought on by poor posture, which is frequently brought on by muscular imbalances and stiffness. These imbalances may be redressed, stiff muscles can be lengthened, and posture can be improved through stretching.

Additionally, stretching calls for body awareness and movement awareness, which can improve body awareness and make you feel more connected to your body. This improved proprioception, or the capacity to feel where your body is in space, can lead to better balance, coordination, and body awareness.

It's crucial to be aware that there are various kinds of stretching, including proprioceptive neuromuscular facilitation (PNF) stretching, dynamic stretching, and static stretching. It's crucial to select the best sort of stretching for your needs and objectives because each has advantages and is appropriate for certain circumstances.

 To prevent damage, stretching should always be done sensibly and within your capabilities. When stretching, the muscles should be warmed up and the stretch should not be painful or uncomfortable. Before including stretching in your regimen, it is advisable to speak with a healthcare provider or certified fitness instructor if you have any pre-existing medical ailments or concerns.

In conclusion, stretching is a crucial component of a healthy lifestyle and has many advantages for both your physical and mental health. It can lower the risk of injuries and encourage relaxation while enhancing flexibility, circulation, posture, and body awareness. Including customary

Examples of Warm-up Exercises

The pelvic floor, back, and abdominal muscles make up the core muscles, which are essential for supporting the spine, preserving balance, and enhancing posture. Regular core workouts can increase functional mobility in seniors, lower the risk of falls, and improve daily activities including bending, lifting, and twisting.

This post is meant to help if you're a novice seeking to start a regular workout regimen. We'll look at many gentle and efficient core exercises made especially for seniors, with a focus on accessibility and safety.

These introductory core exercises can help you lay a strong foundation for a healthy and active lifestyle, whether you're new to fitness or hoping to keep your physical strength as you age. So let's begin your journey to a more powerful and stable core!

Chapter 3

Beginners Core Exercises

Building a strong core is vital for overall fitness and stability. In this post, we'll cover easy and effective core workouts suited for beginners to launch their fitness journey.

Basic exercises for seniors with limited mobility

1. Sitting Marching

Place your feet flat on the ground while sitting comfortably on a comfortable chair. One knee should be raised to your chest and then brought back down. After that, do the opposite knee. Improved leg strength, joint mobility, and circulation are all benefits of this workout.

2. Leg raises while seated

Sit on a chair with your feet flat on the floor and your back straight. Slowly extend one leg in front of you before bringing it back down. the other leg, and repeat. This workout strengthens the lower body by concentrating on the thigh muscles.

3. Chair yoga

Sit on a chair with your feet flat on the floor and perform chair yoga. Practice mild yoga postures such as shoulder rolls, sitting twists, and neck stretches. Strength, relaxation, and flexibility are all enhanced by chair yoga.

4. Row while seated

Sit in a chair with your feet flat on the floor to row while seated. Pulling your elbows back towards your chest and then extending them forward can help you mimic the motion of rowing while holding onto the chair's sides. This workout strengthens your upper body by working your back, shoulders, and arms.

5. Seated shoulder press.

Sit in a chair with your feet flat on the floor and perform a seated shoulder press. Hold a water bottle or a light dumbbell at shoulder height in each hand. Lift the weights straight up into the air and then immediately lower them again. This workout strengthens your upper body while focusing on your shoulders.

6. Ankle circles

Sit in a chair with your feet just off the floor and perform ankle circles. Your ankles should be rotated in a circle, first in one direction and then the other. This exercise enhances circulation and flexibility in the ankles.

7. Hand grip

Sit in a chair with your feet flat on the floor and perform the hand grip exercise. Squeeze as hard as you can for a few seconds while holding a softball or a hand grip tool in your hand, then let go. This exercise strengthens the grip and hands.

8. Seated calf raises

Sit in a chair with your feet flat on the floor and perform seated calf raises. As high as you can, slowly raise your heels off the ground, then slowly bring them back down. This workout strengthens the lower legs by working the calf muscles.

9. Seated hip marches

Sit in a chair with your feet flat on the floor and perform seated hip marches. Lift one foot off the ground slightly and march in place. Then, bring that foot back to the floor and repeat with the other foot. This exercise helps increase leg strength and hip mobility.

10. Seated chest press

Sit on a chair with your feet flat on the floor and perform a seated chest press. At chest height, hold a light dumbbell or a resistance band in each hand. Bring the weights or band back to your chest after pushing them straight out in front of you. This workout strengthens your upper body while working on your chest.

Note: Before beginning any workout program, it's crucial to speak with a healthcare provider, especially if you have restricted mobility or other pre-existing medical concerns. To prevent damage, start with modest weights or resistance and increase it gradually. Never push through pain or discomfort during exercise; instead, pay attention to your body.

Modifications for Each Exercises

1. Seated Marching Modification

If elevating the knees is problematic, seniors can execute ankle pumps by lifting their heels off the ground while keeping their toes on the floor. This can still aid improve circulation and leg mobility.

2. Seniors can start with lesser leg motions, such as lifting their feet just a few inches off the ground instead of fully raising their legs, when performing seated leg raises. If

necessary, they can also cling to the chair's sides for support.

3. Seniors can undertake modest seated stretches and motions within their comfortable range of motion by modifying chair yoga. For additional support while striking postures, they can also employ props like a folded blanket or bolster.

4. Seniors can modify seated rowing by using resistance bands or tubing fastened to the chair's sides rather than pulling on the chair itself, if one is available. For weaker people, this may offer a kinder resistance.

5. Seniors might start with lesser weights or no weights at all and concentrate on controlled motions when performing the seated shoulder press modification. If it's easier on their shoulders, they can also

execute the exercise with their hands
facing inward.

6. Seniors who find it difficult to circle their
   ankles can reduce the size of the circle or
   only flex and extend their ankles. They
   should only move as far as they can
   without experiencing pain.

7. Seniors can modify their hand grip
   exercises by using a stress ball or softball
   and varying the amount of pressure they
   apply to the object. To increase hand
   mobility, they can also do stretches and
   opening exercises.

8. Seniors can modify seated calf raises by
   elevating their heels just a little bit off the
   floor or by simply pressing their toes into
   the ground to engage the calf muscles.

9. Seated Hip Marching Modification:
   Seniors who find it difficult to elevate
   their feet might tap their feet on the floor

in a marching motion or execute smaller, slower hip marches.

10. Seniors can modify the seated chest press by using smaller weights or resistance bands and modifying the range of motion to fit their comfort level. For increased stability, they can also carry out the exercise while holding onto one handle or grip with both hands.

Seniors should always pay attention to their bodies, begin with exercises suited to their level of fitness, and go at their own pace. To ensure the workouts are safe and effective, it is always advised to speak with a healthcare provider or certified fitness instructor.

Advice on correct posture and technique

Keep a decent posture by sitting up straight, keeping your shoulders down, and supporting your back. Maintaining appropriate posture and reducing strain on your back and neck when completing sitting workouts need you to avoid slouching or hunching over.

1. Start Slowly and Gradually

As your strength and level of comfort improve, gradually up the intensity by starting with mild motions and light resistance. Avoid fast or jerky movements that could put stress on your joints or muscles.

2. Control Your motions

Keep your emotions flowing and under control as you do each exercise. Avoid using momentum or swinging when executing the exercises; instead, engage the muscles that are being worked on and move slowly.

3. Respect Your Range of Motion

Only move within your range of motion that is pain-free. Don't stress your muscles or joints past what is comfortable for them. Stop exercising and make appropriate changes if you encounter any pain or discomfort.

4. Use Proper Breathing Technique

When executing the exercises, maintain your breathing regular and natural. Holding your breath can cause your blood pressure to rise and your muscles to grow sore. During the easier section of the workout, inhale, and during the more challenging portion, exhale.

5. Use the right tools

If you're using weights or resistance bands, pick proper resistance levels that will keep you on your toes without placing too much strain on you. Make that the equipment is in perfect operating order and is utilized safely, conforming to any instructions or recommendations supplied.

6. Focus on Balance and Stability

If balance is a problem, do exercises while sitting on a stable chair or with support from a solid surface, like a wall or a countertop. To guarantee stability, employ handrails or other supports as necessary.

7. Take Note of Your Body

Pay close attention to how your body feels while exercising and afterward. Stop exercising and take a break if you experience any pain, discomfort, or dizziness. Consult a medical specialist if your symptoms don't go away.

8. Stay hydrated

Drink water to be appropriately hydrated before, during, and after exercise, especially if you have any medical issues that may call for more fluid intake.

9. Seek skilled Advice

To make sure you are exercising safely and successfully, consider receiving advice from a competent fitness professional or healthcare

practitioner if you are new to exercise or have
any health issues.

When starting any training program, safety
should always come first, especially for senior
people with limited mobility. Always pay
attention to your body, start with workouts that
are good for your level of fitness, and receive
advice from a professional if necessary.

Chapter 4

Intermediate Core Exercises

For comprehensive functional fitness and quality of life as we age older, maintaining a strong and stable core is vital. Our posture, balance, and daily actions like bending, lifting, and twisting are all supported by the core, which is made up of the muscles in the abdomen, lower back, and pelvis.

Regular core exercises can help seniors achieve more stability, balance, and core strength, which can increase their independence and minimize their danger of falling and getting hurt.

We will cover intermediate core exercises in this chapter that are created especially for seniors who have previously acquired a base of core strength through basic exercises. These more advanced exercises are meant to subject the core muscles to new demands, encouraging the development and strengthening of the core muscles. For seniors looking to increase their core training, these exercises can be included in a well-rounded fitness plan with the appropriate form and technique.

Seniors should speak with their healthcare provider before beginning any new exercise program to make sure they are physically prepared and to go over any particular considerations or modifications that could be required. To prevent harm, it's also vital to pay attention to your body, start at a level appropriate for your fitness level, and increase gradually. Let's explore the world of intermediate core exercises for seniors now and find out how they can boost your physical health.

Exercises that are Challenging for seniors with some experience

1. Medicine Ball Slams

A rather light medicine ball can be utilized for 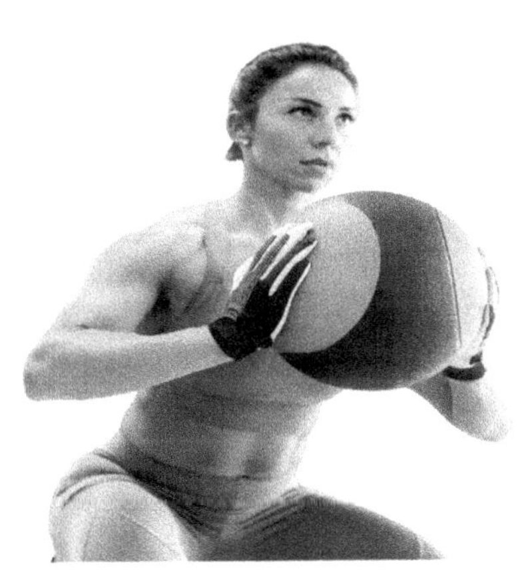 this activity. The senior should hold the medicine ball above their head while standing with their feet shoulder-width apart. Then, while stooping and concentrating on their core and upper body, they should violently slam the ball to the ground. Enhancing balance, upper body strength, and core strength are all benefits of this workout.

2. Single Leg Deadlifts

This lower body workout tests stability and balance while also working the upper body. The senior should take a tall stance with their feet hip-width apart, slowly hinge forward from the hips, elevate one leg in the air, and extend the opposing hand toward the ground. Once back at the 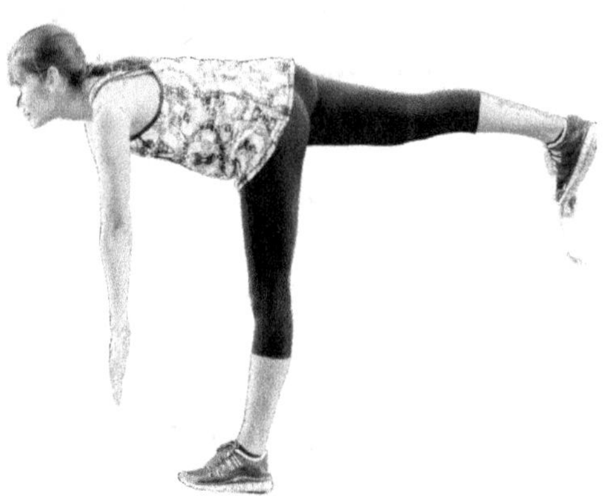 initial spot, they should repeat on the opposing side. This exercise focuses on the core, glutes, and hamstrings.

3. Plank with Leg Lifts

This exercise combines leg lifts to increase the difficulty of a normal plank. With their forearms on the ground and their bodies in a straight line, the senior should begin in a plank stance. Then, while still retaining a firm plank posture, they

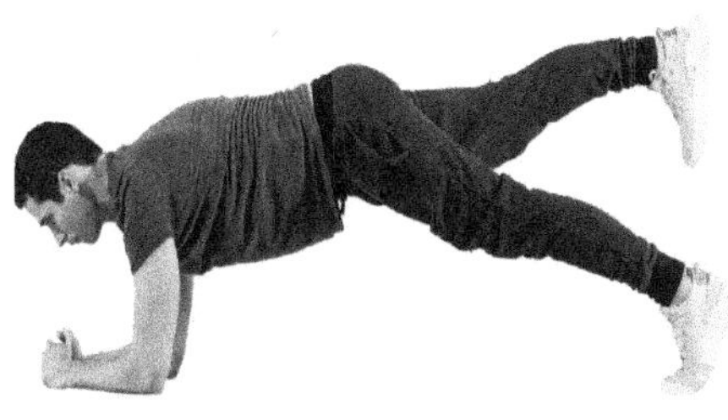

should raise one leg off the floor and lower it back down. They can lift a specified number of times on each leg or alternate legs. The core, shoulders, and glutes are all strengthened by this workout.

4. Rows with a resistance band

The seniors can enhance their upper body

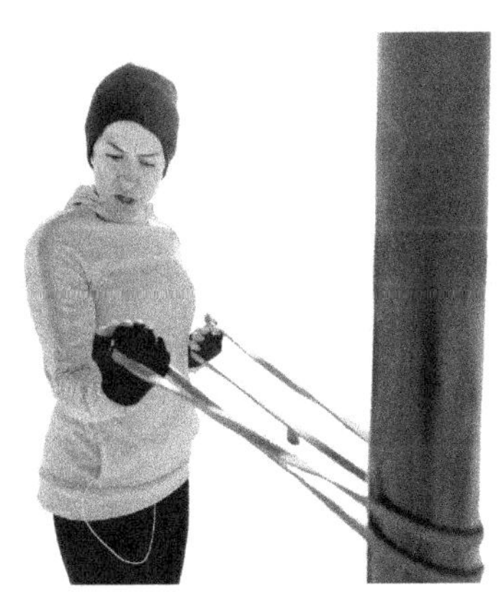

strength by utilizing a resistance band. After attaching the resistance band around a solid object at waist level, they should take a step back to tighten the band. They should draw the band towards their body while keeping their feet shoulder-width apart and pushing their shoulder blades together. This workout focuses on the shoulders, biceps, and back muscles.

5. Step-Ups with Knee Drive

This exercise tests the coordination, balance,

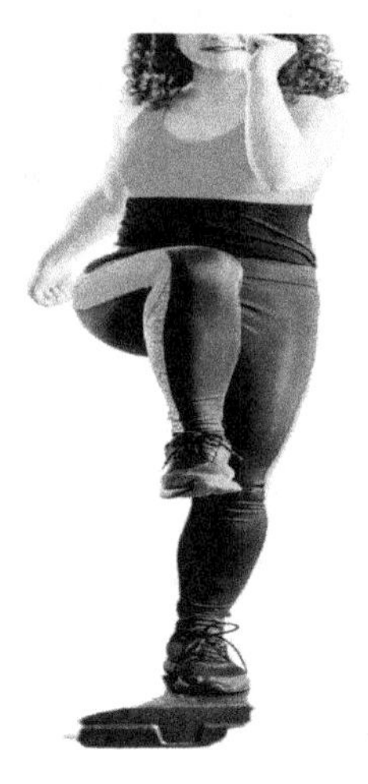

and strength of the lower body. Finding a firm step or platform, the senior should clamber up onto it with one foot while bringing the other knee up toward their chest. After that, they should descend once more and repeat on the opposite side. The quadriceps, glutes, and core are the focus of this exercise.

6. Tricep Dips with Leg Extension.

This workout focuses on the triceps, core, and

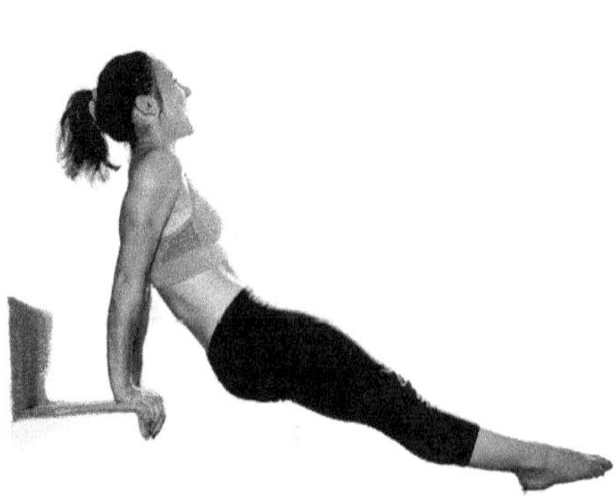

lower body. Tricep Dips with Leg Extension. The senior should take a seat on a sturdy chair or bench with their fingers pointing forward and their hands resting on the edge of the seat. After that, they should stretch one leg straight out in front of them while lowering their chest toward the ground while bending their elbows. Pushing back up to the starting position, they should then switch to the other leg and repeat. Leg strength, core stability, and upper body strength are all put to the test with this workout.

Note: Before starting any new exercise program, seniors should talk with their healthcare physician or a trained fitness expert. They should also start with weights and resistance levels that are suitable for their experience level and degree of fitness. When exercising, safety and excellent technique should always come first.

Modifications for Each Exercises

1. Medicine Ball Slams

If employing a medicine ball is too tough for seniors, they may start with a smaller and lighter weighted ball, such as a soft sand-filled ball or a tiny pillow, and gradually add power as they go.

Seniors with mobility limitations may perform seated medicine ball slams by sitting on a firm chair, gripping the ball in both hands, and slamming it down toward the floor.

2. Single Leg Deadlifts

Seniors with balance concerns may execute this exercise while supporting themselves by grasping onto a strong surface, such as a chair or countertop.

Seniors may start with a restricted range of motion or keep their toes lightly touching the ground for extra support if lifting one leg behind them is too challenging.

3. Plank with Leg Lifts

Seniors may alter this exercise by completing it on their knees while keeping a strong core and lifting one leg at a time if a complete plank posture is too taxing.

To relieve the pressure on their upper bodies, seniors with weak wrist or shoulder muscles could finish the exercise with their forearms resting on an elevated surface, such as a bench or step.

4. Resistance Band Rows

Seniors with weak grips could utilize the handles or loops that are fastened to the resistance band for a more stable hold.

Seniors may do seated rows by sitting on a solid chair with the band secured around their feet and drawing the band towards their chest if standing and pulling the band towards the body is too difficult.

5. Step-Ups with Knee Drive

Seniors who struggle with balance or coordination should start with a lower step height or seek aid from a firm chair or railing.

Seniors may undertake a shortened version if raising the knee towards the chest is too difficult by lifting the knee just as high as is comfortable or by simply stepping up onto the platform without the knee drive.

Seniors with weak upper body muscles may do tricep dips with bent knees by putting their feet on the ground and focusing on the leg extension action.

6. Tricep Dips with Leg Extension.

Seniors who find it difficult to dip to the floor might perform a partial dip with a restricted range of motion or raise their upper body on a sturdy chair or bench to decrease the pressure on their triceps.

Seniors should continually pay attention to their bodies, begin with the correct modifications, and move at a speed that appears secure and comfortable to them.

Before beginning any new training plan, it is important to talk with a healthcare professional or trained fitness expert.

Advice on optimal posture and technique

For safe and effective exercise, particularly for the elderly, appropriate form and technique are necessary. Following are some recommendations for retaining optimal shape amid the hard tasks indicated earlier:

1. Medicine Ball Slams

Maintain a neutral spine and a firm core while standing with your feet shoulder-width apart.

- To produce power, utilize your whole body; don't put too much tension on your lower back.

- Avoid bending or rounding the back as you smash the ball to the ground; instead, focus on making a purposeful, forceful move.

2. Single Leg Deadlifts

Maintain a modest bend in the knee of the supporting leg while maintaining the back straight and hanging from the hips.

- Avoid rotating the hips or shoulders while maintaining the lifted leg in line with the torso.
- Focus on balance and stability throughout the exercise while utilizing your core.

3. Plank with Leg Lifts

Starting in a solid plank posture with the hands or forearms shoulder-width apart and the body aligned from the head to the heels, practice leg raises.

- Avoid allowing the hips or lower back to slump by maintaining core stability.

- Lift one leg at a time while retaining a solid plank posture and minimizing hip or shoulder rotation or movement.

4. Resistance Band Rows

When executing resistance band rows, maintain your shoulders pushed back and down and avoid slouching or rounding your shoulders.

- Keep your core engaged and try not to lean back too much.
- Concentrate on controlled movements while taking deep breaths as you draw the band closer to the body and press the shoulder blades together.

5. Step-Ups with Knee Drive

Step up utilizing the complete foot, avoiding letting the heel dangle over the edge of the step or platform.

- Throughout the whole workout, keep a firm core and a straight back.
- Maintaining stability and balance while pushing the knee toward the chest.

6. Tricep Dips with Leg Extension

On a stable surface, maintain your hands shoulder-width apart and lower your body carefully to avoid placing too much stress on your shoulders.

- Avoid allowing the shoulders or hips to rise toward the ears and maintain your core engaged.
- Legs should be completely extended or you may execute a modified version with bent knees, but make sure the motion is controlled and flowing.

Starting with weights, resistance levels, and adaptations that are suitable for the person's experience level and degree of fitness is vital. If extra information is needed on the right form and technique for safe and effective exercise, contact a healthcare physician or qualified fitness expert may assist.

Chapter 5

Higher Level Core Exercises

A healthy and functional body is founded on a robust and stable core. It is vital for spinal support, retaining good posture, and facilitating optimal movement during everyday chores and sports performance. Although conventional core workouts like crunches and planks are important, there is a range of more demanding core exercises that may boost your core health.

These exercises give a full and well-rounded approach to core training since they stimulate both the deeper stabilizing muscles of the core as well as the superficial abdominal muscles. In this piece, we'll dig into the realm of advanced core exercises, which concentrate on the abs, obliques, lower back, and hips, among other regions of the core.

These advanced routines will push your core training to new heights whether you're an athlete aiming to better your performance or someone looking to improve your general core strength and stability.

Exercises That necessitate a high degree of fitness for the Elderly.

1. Plyometric Step-Up
In this exercise, you step explosively up onto an elevated platform like a solid box or bench. As you progress, gradually increase the height you start at. Power, balance, and coordination in the

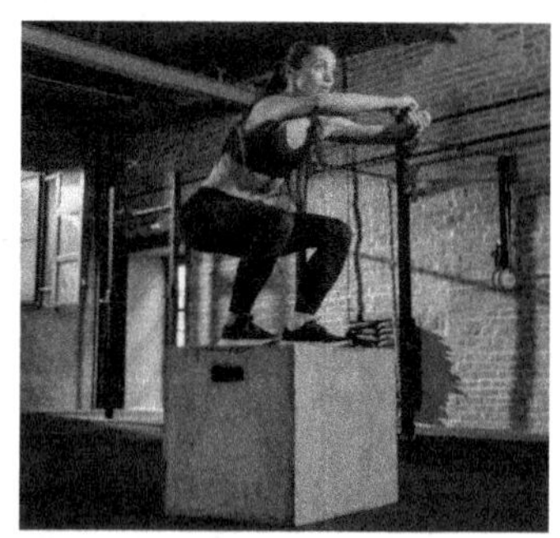

lower body are all strengthened by this training.

2. Dumbbell single-leg deadlift

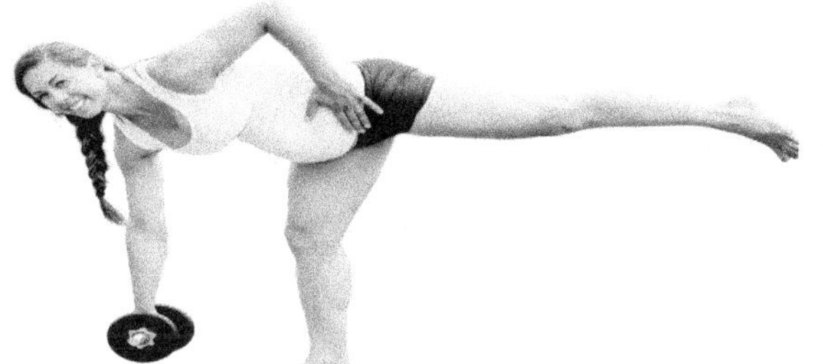

Stand on one leg with the other leg stretched behind you while grasping a pair of dumbbells. While keeping a straight back and a firm core, descend the dumbbells toward the floor, then stand back up. This exercise stresses your balance and stability while exercising your hamstrings, glutes, and core.

3. Swiss Ball Pike exercise.

Starting in a push-up posture with your feet on a Swiss ball, practice the Swiss Ball Pike exercise. While

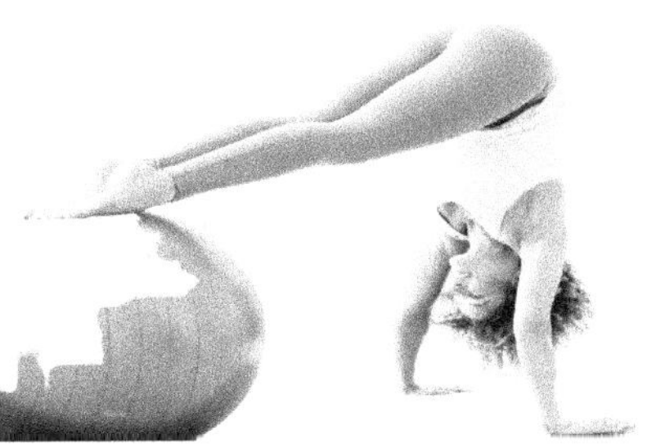

bringing the Swiss ball toward your chest, tighten your core and move your hips upward. Repeat multiple times, lowering yourself back to the beginning position. This exercise challenges your balance and stability while building your core, shoulders, and upper body.

4. Medicine Ball Slams

Lift a medicine ball overhead while holding it in

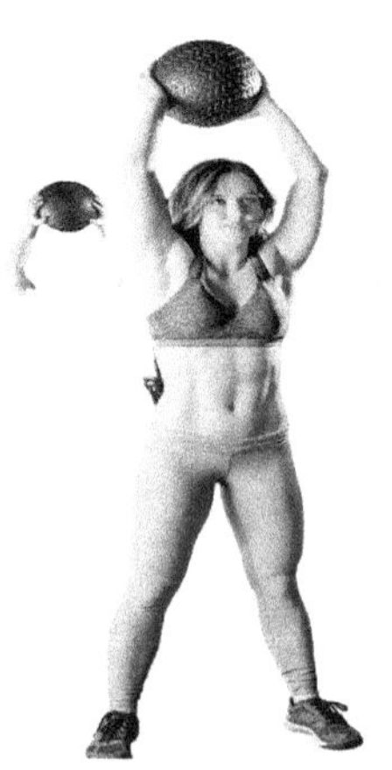

both hands. As hard as you can, smash the ball to the ground, grab it when it bounces back, and repeat it many times. Strength, power, and aerobic fitness in the upper body may all be enhanced with this program.

5. Rotations with a standing resistance band

Stand with your feet shoulder-width apart and a resistance band fastened at chest height. Rotate your body away from the anchor point while gripping the resistance band in both hands. Then, carefully return to the initial position. This exercise stresses your stability and coordination while

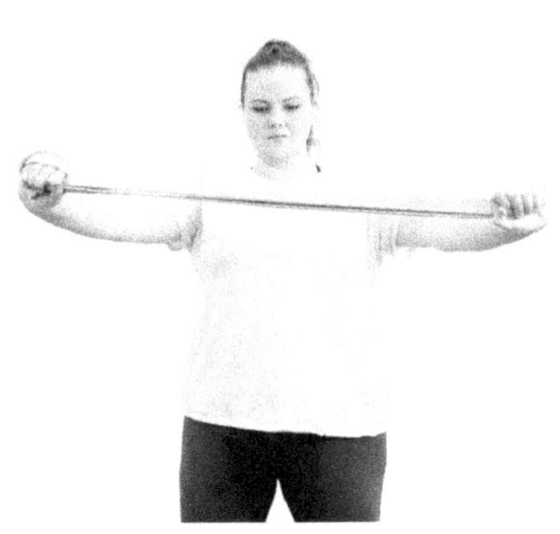

building your core, obliques, and upper body.

6. TRX rows

Setting up a TRX suspension trainer at waist level, standing facing the anchor point, and executing TRX rows. With your arms spread, lean back. Next, bend your elbows and press your shoulder blades

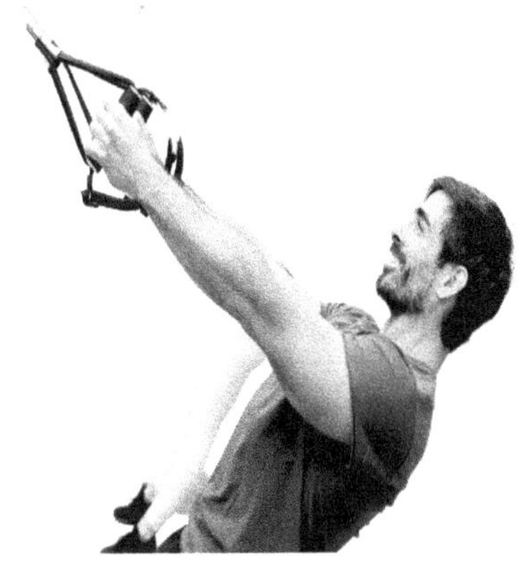

together to pull your body nearer the anchor point. Repeat multiple times, lowering yourself back to the beginning position. The back, arms, and core are all worked out with this exercise, which also measures grip strength and stability.

Note: Before starting any new exercise regimen, it's crucial to consult with a professional fitness expert or healthcare practitioner, particularly if you have any existing medical issues or concerns. They may give precise recommendations and ensure that the routines are suited to your talents and fitness level. Always put safety first and pay attention to your body while exercising.

Modifications for Each Exercises

1. **Plyometric Step-Ups**

To adapt, start with a lower platform height or use a sturdy surface like a staircase instead of a box or bench.

- Reduce the speed and power of the movement to decrease the impact and intensity.
- Hold onto a support, such as a wall or railing, for added stability if needed.

2. Single Leg Deadlifts with Dumbbells

If the balance is an issue, execute the exercise with your back foot softly touching the ground for support.

- Use lighter dumbbells or no weights at all, and gradually increase the weight as you gain strength and stability.
- Perform the exercise on a stable surface, like a flat floor, and avoid using a raised platform.

3. Swiss Ball Pike

Place your hands on a raised surface, such as a bench or step, instead of the ground to lessen the range of motion and intensity.

- Start with a smaller Swiss ball or use an inflatable cushion for added stability.
- Perform the exercise with bent knees to decrease the demand on the core muscles.

4. Medicine Ball Slam

Use a lighter medicine ball or a soft weighted ball if required.

- If slamming the ball onto the ground is too intense, perform an overhead press or a standing Russian twist with the medicine ball instead.
- Engage your core and use your legs to generate power while slamming the ball to reduce strain on the upper body.

5. Standing Resistance Band Rotations

Adjust the resistance of the band by altering the distance from the anchor point or using a lighter band.

- Perform the exercise with a lower range of motion and progressively expand as you build stability and strength.

- Use a wider stance for increased stability or perform the exercise in a seated position if needed.

6. TRX Rows

Adjust the angle of your body by stepping closer or further away from the anchor point to alter the resistance.

- If utilizing a TRX suspension trainer is not possible, practice seated rows with weights or resistance bands.
- Use a wider foot stance or keep your feet on the ground for greater support, and gradually continue to a more challenging posture.

Note: *Remember to continually listen to your body and choose the proper adaptations that suit your fitness level and ability. It's vital to start at a level that is safe and comfortable for you and develop gradually as you build strength and confidence. Consulting with a certified fitness*

Tips for optimal form and Techniques

Proper form and technique are crucial for boosting the efficacy of exercises and lowering the risk of injury, particularly for seniors with advanced fitness levels. Here are some guidelines for retaining adequate form and technique throughout the complex workouts indicated earlier:

1. Plyometric Step-Ups

Keep your core engaged and keep an erect posture throughout the activity.

- Step onto the platform with your complete foot, and avoid having your heel hang off the edge.
- Use a controlled, forceful movement to step up, then softly land with a slight bend in your knees.

2. Single Leg Deadlifts with Dumbbells

Keep your back straight and shoulders pulled back throughout the exercise.

- Hinge at the hips and retain a tiny bend in your standing knee.
- Lower the dumbbells towards the ground in a gradual and controlled way, then engage your glutes and hamstrings to return to the standing posture.

3. Swiss Ball Pike

Start with a plank stance with your hands right under your shoulders and your core engaged.

- Keep your body in a straight line as you elevate your hips towards the sky, and avoid letting your lower backdrop.
- Use your core muscles to regulate the movement and avoid using momentum.

4. Medicine Ball Slams

Hold the medicine ball with a tight grip and use your full body to generate power, including your legs, core, and upper body.

- Keep your feet shoulder-width apart and your knees slightly bent.
- Slam the ball onto the ground with control, and collect it on the rebound with a soft landing.

5. Standing Resistance Band Rotations

Keep your feet shoulder-width apart and your core engaged.

- Rotate your torso away from the anchor point using a controlled and smooth action.
- Avoid excessive twisting of the lower back and preserve the adequate alignment of the spine during the exercise.

6. TRX Rows

Keep your body in a straight line from head to heels, and engage your core to maintain stability.

- Pull your body towards the anchor point by bending your elbows and pulling your shoulder blades together.

- Lower your body back to the starting position in a calm manner, and avoid swinging or arching your back.

In addition to these guidelines, it's crucial to start with sufficient weight or resistance that allows you to maintain perfect form throughout the workout. If you're worried about your form or technique, try working with a skilled fitness professional who can provide feedback and assistance to ensure you're completing the exercises correctly and safely. Always listen to your body, and stop immediately if you experience pain or discomfort during any workout.

Chapter 6

Tips for Progression and Consistency

Core exercises, which target the muscles in your belly, back, and pelvis, are vital for seniors to enhance balance, stability, and general functional fitness. However, it's not just about completing core workouts, but also advancing and being persistent with them to attain the best benefits.

In this chapter, we will cover suggestions for seniors to effectively progress and maintain consistency during core workouts. Whether you're new to core exercises or trying to increase your current regimen, these recommendations can help you optimize your workouts and promote your long-term health and well-being.

Let's dive in and reveal the secrets to successful core workout growth and consistency for seniors!

How to progress to harder exercises

Exercise offers a plethora of benefits for elders, including improved cardiovascular health, increased muscle strength and flexibility, better balance and coordination, and enhanced mental well-being. Engaging in regular physical activity can also help prevent chronic diseases and retain independence in everyday tasks.

As seniors become more comfortable with their exercise routine, it's important to progress to more challenging exercises to continue reaping the benefits and avoid plateauing. Here are some helpful tips on how seniors can progress to more challenging exercises:

1. **Consult with a healthcare professional**
Before starting or progressing to more
challenging exercises, it's crucial to consult with
a healthcare professional, such as a physician or
a certified fitness trainer who has experience
working with seniors. They can assess your
current fitness level, provide personalized
recommendations, and help you set realistic
goals.

2. **Gradual progression**
 It's essential to progress gradually to more
challenging exercises to avoid injuries. Start by
increasing the intensity, duration, or frequency
of your current exercises by a small amount, and
gradually build up over time. For example, if
you're walking for 10 minutes a day, try
increasing it to 15 minutes, and gradually work
your way up to 30 minutes or more.

3. **Incorporate resistance training**
 Resistance training, or strength training, is an
excellent way to challenge your muscles and
bones, and seniors need to maintain muscle mass

and bone density. Start with light weights or resistance bands, and gradually increase the resistance as you get stronger. Resistance training activities can include weight lifting, resistance band exercises, or bodyweight workouts like push-ups, squats, and lunges.

4. Focus on balance and stability

As we age, our balance and stability can decline, increasing the risk of falls. Incorporating exercises that challenge your balance and stability can help improve these skills and reduce the risk of falls. Exercises such as standing on one leg, heel-to-toe walking, or practicing tai chi can be beneficial for seniors. Start with a stable surface, and gradually progress to more uneven or unstable surfaces, such as a balance board or foam pad, to increase the challenge.

5. Try new exercises

Variety is the spice of life, and it's also vital for fitness. Trying new activities may challenge your body in unexpected ways and avoid boredom. For example, if you've been doing largely cardiovascular workouts like walking or cycling, consider trying swimming, dancing, or a group fitness class. If you're accustomed to resistance training with weights, consider utilizing resistance bands or bodyweight workouts to offer diversity and challenge.

6. Don't forget about flexibility

Flexibility exercises are vital for seniors to preserve joint mobility and avoid stiffness. Incorporate stretching exercises into your regimen to increase flexibility. Dynamic stretchings, such as arm circles or leg swings, may be done before exercise to warm up the muscles, while static stretchings, such as touching your toes or shoulder stretches, can be done after exercise when the muscles are warmed up.

7. Listen to your body

It's crucial to pay attention to your body and listen to how it feels during and after exercise. If you experience pain, discomfort, or extreme exhaustion, it may be an indication that you're pushing yourself too hard or executing exercises improperly. It's appropriate to adapt or regress workouts to a more tolerable level or to take rest days as required.

8. Stay hydrated and eat well

Proper hydration and nutrition are critical for seniors to enhance exercise performance and recovery. Drink lots of water before, during, and after exercise, and eat a well-balanced diet that contains protein, healthy fats, and complex carbs to offer the required elements for your body to perform properly.

Importance of constancy in your Regimen during core Exercises

Consistency in routine during core workouts is critical for seniors due to the following major reasons:

1. Muscular Strength and Endurance

Consistent core workouts help seniors gain and maintain muscular strength and endurance. Strong core muscles are needed for stability, balance, and functional movement, which are vital for everyday tasks like walking, standing, and bending.

2. Injury Prevention

Regular core exercises may help seniors lower the risk of falls and injury. A strong core offers stability to the spine and promotes good alignment, lowering the likelihood of accidents and injuries during physical activity.

3. Posture Improvement

Consistent core workouts may help elderly maintain a healthy posture. Poor posture may lead to different difficulties including back discomfort, neck pain, and poor balance. Regular core workouts may help seniors improve their posture and avoid these concerns.

4. Pain Management

Core exercises may be good for seniors suffering from chronic pain disorders, such as lower back discomfort. Consistent core workouts may help strengthen the muscles that support the spine, relieving stiffness and discomfort.

5. Enhanced Balance and Stability

Core workouts concentrate on strengthening the muscles of the abdomen, back, and pelvic area, which play a critical role in maintaining balance and stability. Seniors who frequently undertake core exercises are less likely to incur falls and injuries owing to better balance and stability.

6. Improved Digestion

Core workouts comprise motions that engage the muscles of the abdomen, which may promote digestion and enhance gut health in seniors. Consistently including core exercises in their program may help seniors maintain a healthy digestive tract.

7. Mental Health Benefits

Core workouts, like any other sort of physical activity, produce endorphins, which are mood-boosting chemicals. Consistently exercising in core exercises may help seniors improve their mental well-being, decrease stress, and boost their overall quality of life.

8. **Long-term Health and Independence** Consistency in core workouts may offer long-term health advantages for seniors. Regular core workouts may assist preserve muscular strength, flexibility, and endurance, helping seniors to stay independent and active in their everyday lives.

How to make core workouts a habit

Making core workouts a habit needs regular effort and dedication. Here are some recommendations to help you make core workouts a regular part of your routine:

1. Set Specific Objectives

Define clear and reasonable objectives for your core workouts. It might be increasing the time or intensity of your core exercise, or hitting certain core strength goals. Setting quantifiable objectives can help you remain focused and motivated.

2. Schedule Your Workouts

Treat your core workouts like any other essential appointment and schedule them in your calendar or planner. Set aside concentrated time for your core workouts and make it non-negotiable.

3. Start Small and Progress Gradually

Begin with a reasonable core workout regimen that you can easily include in your everyday routine. Avoid overwhelming oneself with too much too quickly, since this may lead to burnout or damage. Start slowly and progressively increase the length, intensity, or complexity of your core workouts over time.

4. Find Accountability

Share your basic fitness objectives with a workout companion, personal trainer, or a friend who can keep you responsible. Having someone to check in with or work out with might help you keep motivated and on track.

5. Make It Enjoyable

Choose core workouts that you love and that suit your fitness level and preferences. If you find core workouts boring or repetitive, try new kinds of exercises or include diversity into your regimen to make it more pleasurable.

6. Create Reminders

Set reminders or signals to urge you to complete your core workouts. It may be a sticky note on your bathroom mirror, an alarm on your phone, or a calendar notice. Reminders might help you remember to prioritize your core workouts.

7. Be Flexible

Be prepared to alter your core workout regimen to meet changes in your schedule or unforeseen circumstances. It's good to miss an exercise sometimes, as long as you get back on schedule as quickly as possible and don't allow it to impede your overall habit-building success.

8. Reward Yourself

 Celebrate your victories and milestones along the road. Treat yourself to modest pleasures, such as nutritious food, a soothing bath, or some leisure time, after finishing your core workouts. Rewards may reinforce good behavior and push you to continue making core workouts a habit.

Remember, creating a habit takes time and work, so be patient with yourself. Keep persistent, keep concentrating, and ultimately, your core workouts will become a natural part of your everyday routine.

Chapter 7

Common Mistakes and How to Avoid Them

In this chapter, we will analyze several typical errors that people commonly make and give practical recommendations on how to prevent them. From communication mistakes to decision-making errors, we'll dig into major areas where missteps might occur and present solutions for reducing them. Learn from others' errors and boost your chances of success!

Common Mistakes elderly make while practicing core workouts

Core exercises are vital for maintaining strength, stability, and flexibility in the core muscles, which comprise the abdominal muscles, back muscles, and muscles surrounding the pelvis. However, seniors, like any other age group, might make blunders while completing core exercises. Here are some frequent blunders elders may make while practicing core exercises:

1. Poor posture

Seniors may have a propensity to slouch or hunch over when practicing core activities, which may strain the neck, shoulders, and back. It's vital to maintain proper posture throughout the workout, keeping the spine neutral and shoulders relaxed.

2. Overdoing it

Seniors may push themselves too hard, resulting in overexertion or strain. It's vital to start with activities that are suitable for their fitness level and gradually develop over time while listening to their body and avoiding routines that cause pain or discomfort.

3. Holding their breath

Seniors may unwittingly hold their breath when practicing core exercises, which may elevate blood pressure and strain the cardiovascular system. It's crucial to remember to breathe frequently and naturally during the workout, inhaling and exhaling as needed.

4. Neglecting balance and stability

Core workouts need strong balance and stability, and seniors may ignore the relevance of these characteristics. Neglecting balance and stability may lead to falls or injury. It's vital to conduct core exercises on a firm platform and utilize suitable adaptations or support, such as a chair or wall if required.

5. Focusing just on one region

Seniors may tend to concentrate primarily on one section of the core, such as the abs, and ignore other key muscles, such as the back and hips. It's crucial to integrate exercises that target all the main muscle groups in the core for a balanced and effective workout.

6. Rushing through exercises

Seniors may speed through core exercises without paying attention to good form and technique. This may lead to lower efficacy and a greater risk of damage. It's vital to execute core workouts with slow, controlled motions, concentrating on good form and alignment.

7. Not seeking expert help

Seniors may try to practice core exercises without sufficient coaching or supervision. It's vital to contact a trained fitness expert, such as a personal trainer or physical therapist, who can give direction on suitable workouts and adaptations depending on individual requirements and health problems.

Remember, it's always advisable to contact a healthcare physician before beginning any fitness regimen, particularly if you have any underlying health issues or concerns. Proper technique, moderate development, and listening to your body are crucial to safe and successful core workouts for seniors.

How to prevent injuries and setbacks during core workouts for elderly

As we age, it's crucial to exercise and maintain a strong core to promote general health and avoid injuries. However, it's also necessary to be cautious of possible hazards and take measures during core workouts for seniors. Here are some methods to prevent injuries and setbacks:

1. **Consult with a healthcare professional** Before beginning any exercise program, including core exercises, seniors should consult with their healthcare provider to ensure that they are medically cleared for physical activity and to get recommendations on appropriate exercises for their health status.

2. **Warm-up and stretching** Warming up and stretching before participating in core workouts may help avoid injury. Start with a few minutes of modest aerobic exercise,

such as brisk walking, and then execute gentle dynamic stretches for the key muscle groups in the core, such as the lower back, abdominal muscles, and hips.

3. Choose appropriate exercises

Not all core workouts are suited for seniors. Avoid workouts that entail severe bending, twisting, or substantial strain on the neck, lower back, or hips. Opt for exercises that are low-impact and concentrate on stability and balance, such as sitting marches, seated leg lifts, or moderate torso twists.

4. Use good form and technique

Maintaining proper form and technique during core workouts is vital to avoid injuries. Engage your core muscles and move gently and controlled, avoiding abrupt jerking or twisting actions. Use adaptations or props, such as chairs or stability balls, to aid with balance and support as required.

5. Start with low intensity and develop gradually

It's crucial to start with low-intensity workouts and progressively raise the difficulty level as your strength and endurance improve. Avoid overexertion or pushing beyond your limitations, since this might raise the chance of injuries and setbacks.

6. Listen to your body

Pay attention to your body's indications and stop immediately if you experience pain, discomfort, or dizziness during core exercises. Rest and recuperate if you notice any pain or weariness following workout sessions.

7. Stay hydrated and wear suitable gear

Proper hydration is vital for general health and may help reduce muscle cramps and exhaustion during exercise. Wear comfortable and supportive footwear to enhance stability and lessen the chance of slips or falls.

8. Incorporate rest days

Rest days are vital for enabling your body to recuperate and avoid overuse issues. Plan frequent rest days between core training sessions to allow your muscles and joints time to recover and revitalize.

Remember, safety should be the primary issue when core workouts for seniors. Always check with your healthcare practitioner or a competent fitness expert for specific guidance and suggestions based on your unique health state and fitness level.

Tips for overcoming hurdles and remaining on target during core workouts for seniors

Here are some recommendations for overcoming hurdles and remaining on track during core workouts for seniors:

1. Start Slow

It's crucial, to begin with, mild and basic core workouts that suit your fitness level. Avoid pushing yourself too hard and risking damage. Start with easy movements like sitting marches, pelvic tilts, or moderate twists, and progressively develop as you feel comfortable and secure.

2. Listen to Your Body

Pay heed to your body's suggestions throughout the activity. If you encounter pain or discomfort, stop immediately and adapt the workout or see a healthcare expert. It's vital to prioritize your safety and well-being above pushing through pain.

3. Use Proper Form

Proper form is vital for successful and safe core workouts. Follow the recommendations of your exercise instructor or physical therapist to ensure that you are utilizing the right form. Using poor form may lead to ineffective outcomes and increased risk of harm.

4. Adjust workouts

If you have physical limits or health issues, don't be hesitant to adjust workouts to fit your requirements. For example, if you have restricted mobility, you may practice sitting core exercises instead of standing or laying down. Work with your exercise instructor or physical therapist to identify changes that are safe and beneficial for you.

5. Stay Consistent

Consistency is crucial to attaining success. Try to build a regular core fitness plan that you can keep to, whether it's a few times a week or as prescribed by your healthcare expert.

Consistency will help you gain strength and improve over time.

6. Stay Motivated

Staying motivated might be tough, but it's vital for adhering to your basic workout regimen. Find what inspires you, whether it's listening to your favorite music, making personal objectives, or exercising with a buddy. Keep reminding yourself of the advantages of core workouts for your general health and well-being.

7. Stay Hydrated:

Hydration is crucial for any training regimen, particularly core exercises. Make sure to drink enough water before, during, and after your exercise to keep your body hydrated and performing effectively.

8. Rest and recuperate

Don't forget to allow your body ample time to rest and recuperate. Overdoing it may lead to burnout and raise the risk of damage. Listen to your body and take rest days as required to enable your muscles to heal and mend.

9. Seek Professional instruction

If you're new to core workouts or have special health problems, it's advisable to seek professional instruction from a fitness instructor or physical therapist. They can give you the right assistance, changes, and comments to help you remain on track and overcome any challenges.

Remember, it's crucial to contact your healthcare practitioner before beginning any new fitness plan, particularly if you have underlying health issues or concerns. They may give you individualized recommendations based on your unique requirements and help you remain on track with safe and effective core workouts for seniors.

Importance of core strength for overall health

Core strength, which refers to the strength and stability of the muscles in the abdomen, back, and pelvic areas, plays a critical role in general health. Here are some basic reasons why core strength is vital for sustaining overall health:

1. Posture and Spinal Health

A strong core helps maintain excellent posture and supports the spine, which is the major structure of the body. Weak core muscles may lead to poor posture, which can result in greater stress on the spine and contribute to illnesses such as chronic back pain and postural abnormalities.

2. Stability and Balance

Core muscles offer stability and balance to the body during movement and physical activity. Strong core muscles aid in maintaining balance, stability, and coordination, which helps minimize falls and accidents, especially as we age.

3. Functional Fitness

Core strength is crucial for completing daily movements such as lifting, bending, twisting, and reaching. Whether it's taking up a big item or playing a sport, a strong core helps the body to move effectively and with less chance of injury.

4. Performance in Physical Activities

Core strength is vital for athletes and those interested in physical activities such as sports, weightlifting, and endurance training. It boosts performance by boosting power, agility, and general body control.

5. Preventing and Rehabilitating Injuries

A strong core may help avoid injuries by giving stability to the spine and supporting other joints, such as the hips and shoulders. It may also benefit the healing process after an accident, as strong core muscles help support and protect the afflicted region.

6. Metabolic Health

Core workouts may also activate muscles in the abdomen, helping to burn calories, enhance metabolism, and maintain a healthy weight. A healthy weight and metabolism are crucial components of general health and may help avoid numerous chronic health disorders such as obesity, diabetes, and heart disease.

7. Improved Breathing and Digestion

Core muscles also have a role in breathing and digestion. Strong core muscles aid in the mechanics of breathing and support the diaphragm, which is the major muscle responsible for breathing. Additionally, a strong core may help in normal digestion and ease difficulties such as constipation and bloating.

core strength is crucial for general health and well-being. It plays a key function in maintaining the body's stability, balance, posture, and performance in physical activities, while also assisting in injury prevention, rehabilitation, and metabolic health.

Incorporating regular core strengthening exercises into your workout program may be advantageous for maintaining excellent physical health and quality of life. However, it is always advisable to contact a healthcare practitioner or a skilled fitness trainer before beginning any new exercise program, particularly if you have pre-existing health ailments or concerns.

Tips for adding core workouts into your routine

Incorporating core workouts into your regular regimen may be excellent for improving your posture, stability, and general strength. Here are some recommendations to help you make core workouts a regular part of your everyday routine:

1. Start with a warm-up

Just like any training regimen, it's necessary to warm up your muscles before participating in core movements. You may undertake a few minutes of modest aerobic activity such as brisk walking, cycling, or jumping jacks to get your heart rate up and warm up your muscles.

2. Choose a range of exercise

Many various kinds of core exercises target distinct muscle groups inside the core, such as the rectus abdominis, obliques, transverse abdominis, and back muscles. Incorporate a range of exercises including planks, Russian twists, leg lifts, and bridges to train various portions of your core and keep your practice fresh.

3. Start with the fundamental

If you're new to core workouts, it's recommended to start with the basics and progressively increase as your core strength improves. Exercises like the plank, which can be tweaked to varying degrees of difficulty, are a fantastic beginning point. You may start with shorter lengths and progressively increase the time as you gain strength.

4. Focus on good form

Maintaining proper form is vital for successful core workouts and decreasing the chance of injury. Pay attention to your posture, activate your core muscles, and prevent any jerky movements. If you're uncertain about your form, try working with a skilled fitness expert or physical therapist.

5. Make it a habit

Consistency is crucial when it comes to implementing core workouts into your regimen. Aim to complete core exercises at least 3-4 times a week, and progressively increase the length and intensity as you gain stronger. You may also find creative methods to include core workouts into your regular routines, such as performing standing crunches while brushing your teeth or sitting on an exercise ball while working at your desk.

6.   Listen to your body

Pay attention to how your body feels during and after core workouts. If you encounter pain or discomfort, stop and seek a healthcare expert. It's crucial to listen to your body and not push yourself past your boundaries.

7.   Switch it up

To keep things fresh and avoid monotony, switch up your core workout regimen. Try various workouts, alter the difficulty, and bring in new difficulties as you grow. This might help you remain motivated and continue to build your core strength.

Incorporating core workouts into your routine may have numerous advantages for your overall fitness and health. Remember to start softly, concentrate on perfect form, and be consistent. With time and effort, you may grow a stronger core and experience the advantages of enhanced stability and strength.